# Master Medical Coding with this Comprehensive Guidebook

Ralphie .L Chambers

*Master Medical Coding with this Comprehensive Guidebook : Unlock the Secrets of Medical Coding with this Ultimate Handbook.*

## _Funny helpful tips:_

_Stay informed; knowledge empowers and enlightens._

_Stay vigilant about dental health; regular check-ups and good oral hygiene are essential._

## _Life advices:_

_Avoid making assumptions; seek clarity through conversation._

_Seek recommendations from experts in fields of interest; their insights can guide you to seminal works._

# Introduction

In this book, readers are taken on a comprehensive journey through the world of healthcare, starting with an exploration of the fundamental concepts and components of the field. The book begins by examining healthcare itself, including health insurance and health information, setting the stage for a deeper understanding of healthcare billing and the role of medical billers and coders.

Readers gain insights into both medical billing and medical coding, with a clear distinction between the two. The importance of coding in medical billing is emphasized, shedding light on the vital role it plays behind the scenes. Various types of medical coding are introduced, providing a well-rounded view of this aspect of the profession.

The book then delves into the intricacies of the medical billing process, with an emphasis on the responsibilities of medical billers and coders. Legal aspects, medical terminologies, and procedures are discussed in detail, providing readers with a solid foundation in the field.

Understanding body systems and medical procedures becomes crucial, as readers explore the intricacies of evaluation and management codes. Commercial health insurance and Medicaid billing are examined to provide a comprehensive view of the billing landscape.

For those aspiring to embark on a career in medical billing and coding, the book offers valuable insights into basic certifications and the certification process. Prospective students are guided through the steps to prepare for their studies and certification exams.

The importance of software in medical coding is highlighted, along with an exploration of medical billing contracts, referrals, and prior authorization. Claim tracking and appeal procedures are thoroughly covered, ensuring readers are well-prepared to navigate the complexities of the billing and coding process.

Readers gain a comprehensive understanding of CPT codes, modifiers, claim edits, clearinghouses, and medical reimbursement. Ambulance transportation billing and claim denials are addressed, with a focus on remittance advice and dispute resolution.

The book sheds light on the role of ICD codes and the involvement of payers in the medical billing process, including working with Medicare contractors and understanding Medicare Advantage Plans. It also emphasizes the importance of improving the billing experience for patients, maintaining patient confidentiality, and efficiently collecting patient payments.

To help readers avoid common pitfalls, the book explores common billing and coding mistakes and offers top tips from experts in the field. Throughout the journey, readers gain a deep understanding of the multifaceted world of medical billing and coding, making it an invaluable resource for beginners and those looking to enhance their knowledge in this critical healthcare profession.

# Contents

# CHAPTER ONE A Look at the Concept of Healthcare

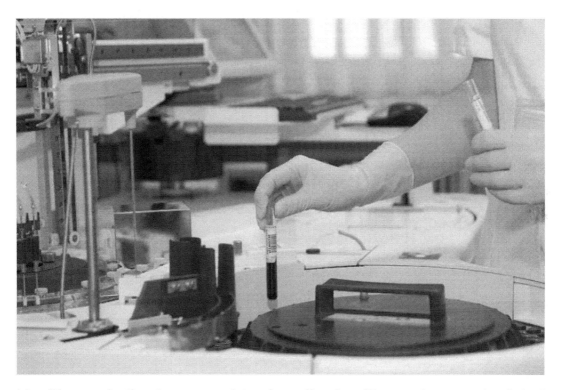

Healthcare is the term used to describe health services and related matters offered by health professionals (physicians, dentists, veterinarians, etc.) or by healthcare institutions (hospitals, clinics, etc.) to patients. The healthcare industry offers healthcare services in the following areas:

## Health Insurance

The healthcare industry offers two types of healthcare insurance coverage: indemnity and no-fault. Indemnity insurance is a policy that reimburses its holder in the event of a health-related claim. For example, if you get sick, a doctor will tell you to pay a certain amount of money for medical services, and you get indemnity insurance to help pay for your medical expenses. If the doctor is wrong and the medical expenses aren't covered, you can then request reimbursement for those expenses.

No-fault insurance pays out directly to its beneficiaries in the event that they suffer a health-related problem that isn't considered being the fault of the healthcare provider.

## Health Information

Healthcare is also known as medical information, health information, and health records. Health information is information that can be used to help patients and physicians manage their health. There are several ways to categorize this information, including the National Health Information Network,

Health Level Seven, the International Classification of Diseases, and others. Health information can be found anywhere from patient visit notes to X-ray images to billing statements. Medical records are also known as medical histories, medical charts, medical records, case notes, patient records, or patient health records.

## Healthcare Billing

Healthcare billing is the process of tracking patient services. Healthcare billing is sometimes referred to as "billing", "recording", or "claims management", but these terms are more commonly used to refer to the specific system used by hospitals and healthcare professionals to manage the claims process, as opposed to the process of billing for services. If you visit the doctor for a check-up, for example, you might have a medical record that will indicate when you came in, who you were with, and what your symptoms were. If you stay overnight, you might also have a medical record that will indicate when you came in, what happened during your stay, what tests were performed, and how long it took the doctor to do the tests.

If you are given a medical procedure, you may have a billing record that indicates what was done, the cost, and the date when you were paid for the procedure. If your provider bills your insurance company, then you will be given a statement that indicates what has been covered, what wasn't covered, and how much you owe. The insurance company will also determine how much they want to pay for the services provided. This will then be paid to the provider who provided the services, and you will be reimbursed for the covered portion of the bill.

Once you've been billed and paid for all your services, the next time you receive a medical bill, the bill will have a line item for "balance due". This balance due amount can be for services you haven't yet been billed for, or it can be for services you've already been billed for, but not paid. If you haven't paid this balance due amount, the provider can take steps to ensure you pay them. Healthcare providers will bill patients or insurance companies for services, and the services can be:

- ☐ Medical-only
- ☐ Hospital services
- ☐ Hospital and medical professional services
- ☐ Outpatient services

Outpatient services include things like visits to the dentist or doctor, x-rays, and prescriptions. Outpatient services aren't usually paid for in full by insurance companies unless they cover out-of-pocket expenses. If you have an inpatient stay, which may include surgery, your hospital stay will be covered by insurance, and you will receive a bill from the hospital. However, if you've already been billed for outpatient services at the time your inpatient stay is completed, you will still receive a bill from the hospital, and the insurance company will reimburse you for those services.

## Insight on Medical Billing

The billing and coding process of medical practice is not an end in and of itself. The medical billing professional (or biller) works with a set of doctors who are treating and delivering care to patients. The physician orders a test, a procedure, or surgery, and the health care provider (a radiologist or nurse) provides the services as specified. The biller, typically a billing coordinator, is the interface between the two physicians.

Medical billing is the process by which health care providers bill the health insurance carriers for services provided to patients. To the patient, these services are free. The health insurance carriers must pay for the services that the doctor provides. Thus, medical billing is really only for the reimbursement of doctors. In today's fast-paced health care delivery environment, doctors typically have a lot on their plates. It takes time and coordination to handle the various bills, insurance documents, pay applications, etc. And the doctors have patients to see, which is their primary responsibility. Their medical billing staff, on the other hand, needs to handle and monitor this administrative overhead.

Medical Billing is the most important task for health care firms that want to gain a better market in the medical world. The reason being this industry provides around 40% of the revenue of any health care firm. Medical billing is an organized and specialized job that assists physicians to bill for the treatment that they have provided to their patients. Medical billing services are usually hired by large and medium hospitals, health care companies, and insurance companies. Medical billing is a process of documentation and billing of all the services that are done for patients. The reason for this is that medical billing records the number of procedures and services that are performed on patients and then they bill patients for their cost.

## Insight on Medical Coding

Medical Coding is the process by which Healthcare Providers such as Physicians, nurses, and hospital employees, convert medical records and observations into a useable code set that is interpreted by the computer software that allows for billing and information retrieval. In order to process the billing system and information retrieval into the coding software, Healthcare Providers use the coding manual. The manual defines all the medical codes the computer will interpret as being medical observations that were recorded in the medical record. The medical observations are converted into medical code names that the billing software and information retrieval software use. Medical codes are the name for how observation was recorded in the medical record and how they are interpreted by the coding software. The medical codes also dictate how to bill and how information is retrieved for the healthcare provider and the insurance company.

Medical Coding and coding manuals are one of the many parts of the process used by the healthcare provider to record medical observations, perform procedures, and ultimately bill the insurance company for the service. In the case of healthcare providers in emergency departments, physicians may be using a flow sheet (a chart with time on one axis and the patient's vital signs on the other) to record the medical observations of a patient. This may include observations of abnormal lab work or blood pressure or other patient symptoms that have been documented in the medical record. The medical observations are then turned into a code name that indicates the medical issue that has been documented. For example, if a patient is experiencing shortness of breath they may be documented with an observation of dyspnea. This observation may be recorded as respiratory distress syndrome (RDS) in the medical record.

## Difference Between Medical Billing and Medical Coding

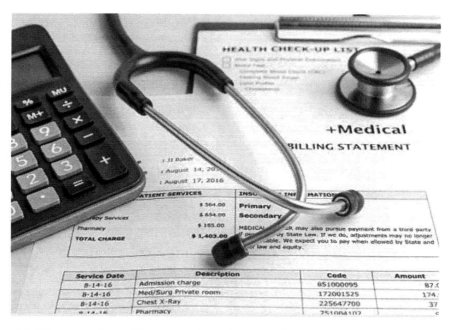

Medical billing and coding are two integral parts of the medical field. They work together to ensure that medical bills are accurate and that insurance companies are billed correctly. However, there are some key differences between the two professions. Medical billing is the process of submitting and following up on claims with insurance companies in order to receive payment for services rendered by a healthcare provider.

Medical coders, on the other hand, take information from doctors' notes, lab reports, and patient charts to assign specific codes to each diagnosis or procedure performed. This code then becomes part of the bill that is sent to an insurance company.

One major difference between these professions is their level of interaction with patients. Medical coders rarely have any contact with patients; their job is mainly administrative. In contrast, medical billers often have face-to-face conversations with patients about their bills and may need to resolve issues or answer questions related to payments."

# CHAPTER TWO Importance of Coding in Medical Billing

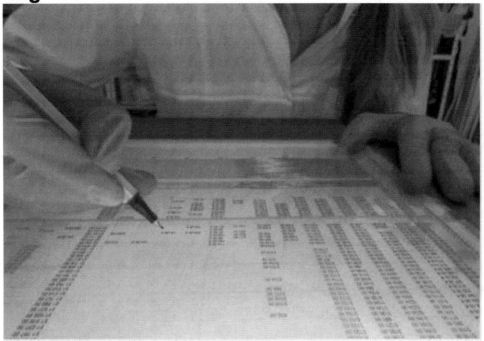

The Coding section of the medical billing process is what sets a provider apart from the rest. As you read this, you should think of your medical biller or the person that handles your coding. If you have an experienced medical biller, then you are in good company. If you have never had to deal with medical coding and billing in your entire medical career, then you should get on it as soon as possible. It is essential that you understand the importance of coding in medical billing and how to do it well.

Coding will always make or break a provider. It is important to remember that medical billing isn't just a money-making tool for medical providers. Medical providers have to think about things such as health care cost, quality of care, patient satisfaction, and how quickly a patient can be seen. They have to balance these various aspects when making decisions on how they are going to bill their patients.

Some medical centers and insurance companies require every visit to be coded and billed in the most efficient manner possible. Other patients don't always understand what is necessary to keep them in good standing with their insurance company. This requires good communication between medical providers and medical billers in order to maximize patient satisfaction. The Coding section is where all the action is. With a medical biller that has great communication skills, the coding section will always come off looking good.

## Behind the Scenes: Medical Billers and Coders

Medical billers and coders are the unsung heroes of the healthcare industry. They work behind the scenes to ensure that medical bills are accurate and processed efficiently. Medical billers are responsible for creating invoices, submitting claims to insurance companies, and following up on payments. They must be knowledgeable about insurance codes and billing procedures in order to ensure that bills are paid correctly.

Coders use these codes to create a billable diagnosis code for each patient visit. This information is used by insurance companies to determine how much they will reimburse healthcare providers for services rendered. Coders must also be familiar with the ICD-10 (the latest version of the International Classification of Diseases) coding system in order to assign the correct code(s) to each patient visit. Both medical billers and coders play a vital role in ensuring that patients receive timely and accurate billing statements for their healthcare services.

## Types of Medical Coding

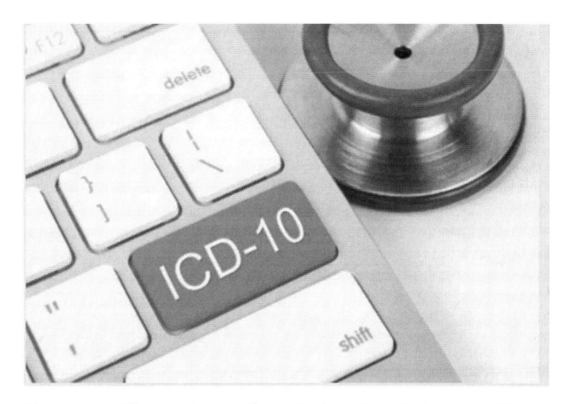

There are different types of medical coding that serve different purposes. If you are a healthcare professional, you need to have an in-depth understanding of all the types of coding that exist. Understanding the different types of medical coding can allow you to get the accurate payments that you deserve. A few very popular types of medical coding are:

**CPT codes**

Codes "CPT" is the acronym of its definition in English, Current Procedural Terminology, commonly known as terminology codes, is a catalog maintained by the American Medical Association through the CPT editorial board. This catalog describes medical, surgical, and diagnostic services in order to unify such information among physicians, coders, patients, institutions, accrediting organizations, and administrators. This unified coding allows for standardizing administrative, financial, and analytical tasks in the sector. The current version of the CPT is CPT 2021.

## HCPCS codes

This type of code, commonly known as "HICK PICS", is a series of medical codes based on the American Medical Association "AMA", currently homologated with the "CPT" codes.

"HCPCS" codes were originally called "HCFA" Common Procedure Coding System, which is the medical billing method used by the Center for Medicare and Medicaid (CMS). Before 2001, this type of medical coding was known as the "HCFA" Health Care Financing Administration, which was established in 1978, in order to provide a standardized form of coding that was capable of specifically describing items and services provided. In the process of medical care. These codes are not used in the Panamanian jurisdiction, and the United States, they are used exclusively for Medicare and Medicaid billing processes to ensure that medical claims are processed in a consistent and standardized manner.

## ICD

The acronym ICD refers to the International Classification of Diseases. It is prepared by the World Health Organization and its international character promotes the creation of global statistics on mortality and morbidity. It is probably the most widespread and one of the most complete coding systems in the health sector. The tenth update, the so-called ICD-10 coding, is currently in use, but the latest version, ICD-11, is expected to appear this year.

## CDT

CDT stands for Current Dental Terminology. In essence, it is very similar to the CPT system already mentioned above, but it has one big difference: this codification of the health sector refers solely and exclusively to oral and dental processes.

Imagine, for example, that you consult diseases related to smoking. The CDT only contemplates those that have to do with the effect of tobacco on the mouth and teeth.

## DSM

The Diagnostic and Statistical Manual of Mental Disorders (DSM) is a classification system for psychiatric illnesses and other disorders, edited by the American Psychiatric Association. As with the CIE, it was created in order to offer a systematic list of codes that all professionals could follow. Over time, mental illnesses ended up being included in the ICD. However, DSM has continued to update at its discretion. The most current version is DSM-V.

# The Process of Medical Billing

The billing and coding team is responsible for ensuring that the proper codes are assigned and that the claims are submitted according to the guidelines set by the government and other payers. The team is also responsible for helping to understand the current rules and regulations surrounding medical billing. The most important step in a medical billing process is that the provider must bill for the service that he or she renders. If there are codes that can be used, the codes should be used. The provider must document the codes in the chart or electronic medical record in a particular way.

The medical billing team is responsible for determining if any questions arise and addressing them. In order to be able to accurately bill for your services and understand what can and cannot be billed, the billing and coding team must be in contact with the patient, including obtaining an electronic medical record (EMR) and obtaining consent forms. This is the time for gathering information from the patient and documenting the pertinent history.

This guide will help you understand the basics of medical billing and how to submit a claim.

The first step in medical billing is to determine which services were provided to the patient. This can be done by reviewing the patient's chart or insurance card. It is important to collect all the information necessary to submit a claim, including:

- ☐ Patient name and address
- ☐ Date of service
- ☐ Provider name and contact information
- ☐ Type of service provided
- ☐ Insurance company name and policy number

Once you have gathered all of this information, you are ready to begin submitting your claim. There are several ways to do this, but most providers use one of two methods: paper claims or electronic claims submission (EDI). Paper claims can be submitted by mail or fax, while EDI uses special software that transmits data electronically between providers and insurance companies. No matter which method you choose, there are some basic elements that every medical bill should include:

- ☐ Patient identification info (name, address)
- ☐ Date(s) services were rendered/provided/ordered/etc.
- ☐ Service codes & descriptions
- ☐ Quantity & unit prices for each code -Total amount charged for all codes
- ☐ Any applicable discounts/adjustments/write-offs etc.

## Understanding your Duty as a Medical Biller/Coder

If you have never taken the time to understand your duty as a medical biller and medical coder, the purpose of this topic is to show you how to do your job better. Not only does it help you understand your professional responsibility, but it may also save your life if you're lucky enough to work for a large health care company where someone is doing their job correctly.

Medical billing and coding is a critical process in the overall healthcare system. It is responsible for accurately recording, classifying, and billing medical procedures and services. This process helps to ensure that healthcare providers are paid correctly for the services they provide, while also helping patients understand their medical bills.

As a medical biller or coder, it is important to understand your duty to both the provider and the patient. Your role is essential in ensuring that all procedures are billed correctly and that patients receive accurate information about their bills. You must also be aware of changes in billing regulations so that you can ensure compliance with these guidelines.

It is also important to maintain a professional attitude at all times when dealing with both providers and patients. Remember that you are representing the entire healthcare industry when you interact with others, so be courteous and respectful at all times. By understanding your role and fulfilling your duties conscientiously, you can help make the billing process more efficient and improve communication between providers and patients.

As a medical biller and coder, you have an important role in the healthcare industry. You ensure that patients receive accurate bills for the services they receive, and you help to ensure that healthcare providers are paid properly for the services they provide.

Your job begins with coding patient visits. This involves assigning codes to each diagnosis and procedure so that bills can be accurately generated. It's important to use the most up-to-date coding system so that claims are processed correctly.

Once visits have been coded by the medical coder, it's your job as a medical biller to submit claim forms to insurance companies on behalf of healthcare providers. You must also follow up on any claims that are denied, in order to determine why they were not paid and work with insurers to get them approved.

In addition, you may be responsible for billing patients directly for out-of-pocket expenses. It's a challenging but essential role in ensuring that patients receive quality care and that providers are fairly compensated for their services.

# CHAPTER THREE Complying with the Legal Aspect of Medical Billingand Coding

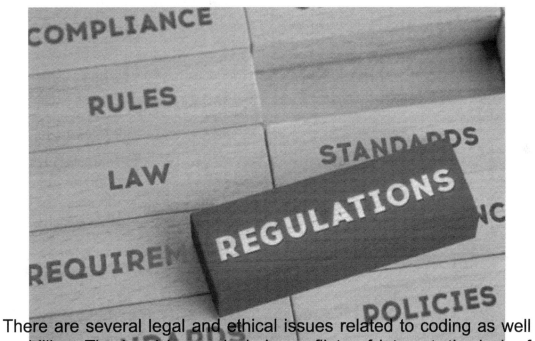

There are several legal and ethical issues related to coding as well as billing. The legal issues include conflicts of interest; the lack of transparency in the coding process; the use of non-medical, non-coding criteria to determine if a service is medically necessary and if it requires additional resources. It may be claimed that the physician is not allowed to have a financial interest in the services provided to the patient, in this case, the physician's services.

However, the physician's legal responsibility also extends to having the financial responsibility for the services provided. As such, to meet their legal and ethical obligations, the physician must also have a financial interest in the services provided to the patient. The physician should be transparent and have full disclosure of the nature and amount of services provided to the patient, as this helps to mitigate the perception of the potential for unethical activity or favoritism, particularly in Medicare and private insurance plans where more scrutiny is applied to the coding of services and the physician's billing.

To meet the ethical aspect of billing and coding, it is important that there is a shared understanding of the code assignment with the physician as to what the code means and to be aware of coding guidelines to ensure the coding is consistent and reflects the professional judgment of the provider. It is also important to recognize the time constraints and pressures placed on physicians, particularly in emergency medicine, to spend adequate time with patients and to bill accurately and effectively.

Health insurance is an important aspect of any health care system and the physician has a duty to obtain authorization and payment for services prior to providing them. It is important to make sure that the patient has insurance coverage for the services provided. This becomes even more important in emergency medicine where the physician is often faced with patients who do not have adequate insurance coverage for the emergency care provided, which can impact the time needed to provide care, as well as the resources necessary to provide the care.

Medical coding and billing is a significant source of income for medical practices, especially those with a large number of patients. Since the practice of medicine is evolving and the reimbursement is being reduced due to the Affordable Care Act (ACA), general practitioners need to be aware of the ACA in order to maintain their practices and stay competitive.

However, billing and coding can also be a source of ethical issues. One issue is physician billing for services that were not provided.

This can include billing for services that were not performed or overbilling for services provided. Another issue is upcoding or charging more than necessary for a service. Upcoding can be done intentionally or unintentionally, but it results in higher costs for patients and taxpayers. There are various laws governing medical billing and coding. These include the Health Insurance Portability and Accountability Act (HIPAA), which sets privacy standards for healthcare information, as well as Medicare coverage guidelines, which specify what services must be covered by Medicare.

In addition, there are state laws that may govern specific aspects of medical billing and coding, such as reimbursement rates or claim submission requirements. It is important for healthcare professionals to be aware of these laws in order to ensure compliance with them when submitting claims for payment. Failing to comply with these laws can result in fines or other penalties imposed by government agencies responsible for enforcing them.

## Understanding Medical Terminologies

There are a lot of medical terminologies used in the medical billing and coding field. It is important to understand these terms in order to accurately bill and code procedures and services. This topic will define some of the most common medical terminologies used in billing and coding. Now let's take a look at some common medical terminology used in billing and coding:

**Diagnosis Code** - A diagnosis code is a three-digit code that represents the principal diagnosis made by the provider during the patient encounter. There are thousands of diagnosis codes available, which can be found in the ICD-10-CM manual.

**Procedure Code** - A procedure code is a four or five-digit code that represents surgical or nonsurgical procedures performed by healthcare providers on patients. There are tens from which procedure codes can be selected.

**HCPCS Level II Codes** - HCPCS level II codes (commonly referred to as "CPT" codes) are five-digit alphanumeric codes that represent outpatient diagnostic tests, laboratory tests, radiologic exams, durable medical equipment (DME), prosthetics/orthotics, and other services not covered under CPT Codes such as ambulance transportation.

**Revenue Code** - A revenue code is a four-digit numeric code used to identify products and services provided by hospitals for reimbursement purposes.

**National Drug Code (NDC)** - The National Drug Code is a unique 11-character identifier assigned to pharmaceuticals marketed in the United States.

**Modifier** - A modifier is two alpha characters appended to multiple procedure codes indicating that a service has been modified from the usual service code(s). For example, "TC" indicates that the procedure was performed with the addition of an endoscope.

**Anatomic pathology** - The study of the structure and function of body tissues, organs, and organ systems.

**Biopsy** - A procedure that removes a small piece of tissue for examination under a microscope.

**E&M services** - Evaluation and management services, which are billed using CPT codes.

**Insurance company** - A business that contracts with healthcare providers to pay for patient care expenses incurred by their members/policyholders.

**Outpatient service** – Healthcare provided outside a hospital setting, such as at a doctor's office or clinic

**Pathology** – The scientific study of disease processes.

**A&P** - Abbreviation for anatomy and physiology. This term is often used when describing the body's various systems and their functions.

**ACO** - Accountable care organization. A type of healthcare organization that is responsible for meeting specific quality metrics in order to earn financial rewards from Medicare or Medicaid. ACOs are also accountable for the costs incurred by their patients.

**CMS** - Centers for Medicare & Medicaid Services. The federal agency that oversees Medicare, Medicaid, and other health insurance programs in the United States. CMS also sets standards for healthcare providers participating in these programs.

There are thousands of modifiers available for these codes, and understanding these terms will help you accurately bill and code procedures and services provided by healthcare providers.

# CHAPTER FOUR Insight on Medical Procedures

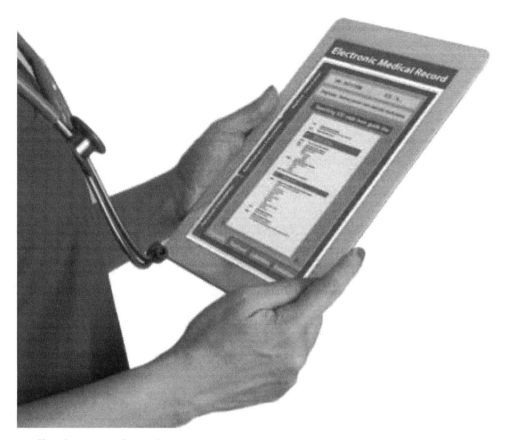

A medical procedure is a planned, usually systematic, and often the invasive treatment of an illness or injury. It may be carried out by a doctor, nurse, or other healthcare professional.

A guide to understanding medical procedures can be extremely helpful for those who are about to undergo one, or for their loved ones. It can provide insight into what to expect before, during, and after the procedure.

Before a medical procedure, it is important to understand why it is being done and what the risks and benefits may be. Ask your doctor any questions you have about the procedure so that you are fully informed. If you are having surgery, be sure to ask your surgeon about his or her experience with the surgery and how often it is performed.

During a medical procedure, you may be given anesthesia so that you will not feel pain. You may also need special equipment such as an IV line or oxygen mask in order to help keep you safe and comfortable. Be sure to let your doctor know if anything feels uncomfortable or if you have any questions during the procedure.

After a medical procedure, it is important to follow your doctor's instructions carefully regarding post-operative care. This may include taking medication prescribed by your doctor, resting as needed, and avoiding certain activities until healing has occurred. By following these guidelines closely, you can ensure a smooth recovery process.

As a medical biller or coder, it is important to understand the procedures that your clinic performs. This will help you code them correctly and ensure that the bills are accurate. It can also help you troubleshoot any billing issues that may arise.

Each procedure has a specific code that is used to identify it. These codes are updated annually by the American Medical Association (AMA) in their CPT manual. You should become familiar with these codes and use them when billing insurance companies or patients.

There are three main types of medical procedures: diagnostic, therapeutic, and surgical. Diagnostic procedures are used to diagnose illnesses or conditions, therapeutic procedures treat illnesses or conditions, and surgical procedures remove organs or tissue.

Some common diagnostic procedures include x-rays, MRIs, and CT scans. Common therapeutic procedures include chemotherapy and radiation therapy treatments. Common surgical procedures include mastectomies and heart bypass surgeries.

It is important to note that not all medical procedures will be billed using CPT codes. There are other billing codes such as HCPCS Level II Codes which can be used for certain outpatient services such as lab tests, durable medical equipment (DME), and ambulance transportation. As a medical biller or coder, it is important to stay up-to-date on all the latest coding changes so that you can accurately bill for the services your clinic provides.

## Aspects of Surgical Procedures

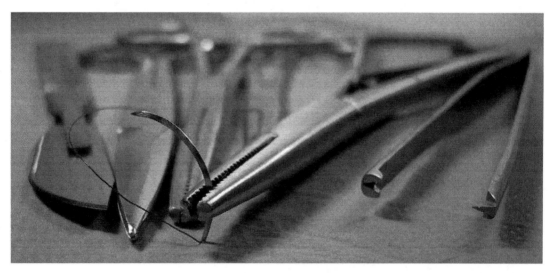

A surgical procedure is a medical treatment that involves making an incision in the body to treat an illness or injury. Surgical procedures can be performed with a variety of instruments, including scalpels, scissors, and lasers. Some common surgical procedures include:

**C-section:** A cesarean section is a surgery used to deliver a baby through an incision in the mother's abdomen.

**D&C:** A dilation and curettage (D&C) is a procedure used to remove tissue from the uterus. It may be done for various reasons such as heavy bleeding or cancer.

**Laparoscopy:** A laparoscopy is a surgery that uses a thin tube with a light and camera on it (a laparoscope) to look inside the abdominal cavity. It may be used to diagnose problems or help guide during other surgeries.

As a medical coder, you may be required to code surgical procedures. While there is no one-size-fits-all guide to coding surgical procedures, there are some general tips that can help make the process easier.

First and foremost, always consult the official CPT manual when coding surgery. This resource is published by the American Medical Association (AMA) and contains all the officially recognized CPT codes for surgical procedures. It's also important to be familiar with modifier usage when coding surgery. Modifiers can be used to indicate specific details about a procedure, such as whether it was performed on an inpatient or outpatient basis.

When coding surgery, it's also important to remember that not all procedures are billed under CPT codes. Some surgeries may be billed using HCPCS Level II codes instead. HCPCS Level II codes are used for services and supplies that aren't covered under CPT but are still considered medically necessary. As a medical coder, it's your responsibility to know which code set should be used for each procedure you encounter. Finally, always remember to use appropriate modifiers when billing for surgery.

## Understanding Body Systems

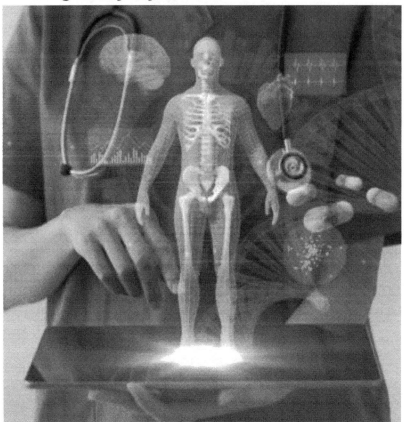

Body systems (BS) are one of the most common terms in medical billing. But how do you know which BS will apply to the patient's health condition? The answer is that you'll have to understand which body system applies to your client and his/her diagnosis, whether it's a code or modifier in the third-level diagnosis.

Understanding the BS terminology and how they're commonly used is very important. Once you know, you can easily code any of the body systems and get reimbursed. To understand BS in coding and medical terminology, it's best to have a basic understanding of what BS are and how they work in medical coding.

# What are body systems?

Your body consists of different organs, tissues, and cells, and they act together to work towards the sustenance of your body and health. However, it's not possible to discuss the various body systems without some knowledge of anatomy. Anatomy is the study of the structure and form of the body, while anatomy goes into the structures of the human body like the bones, joints, tendons, nerves, and muscles. All the different parts of the body are attached and form the different body systems.

In the medical billing environment, we use BS terms quite often in some or all aspects of coding. For example, if the patient has diabetes, he might have problems with blood pressure, eyes, or kidneys. These are the areas that might need treatment and might require attention. Similarly, if a doctor diagnoses any of the above conditions, the doctor may use the corresponding BS codes for treatment, procedures, and medicines.

Understanding body systems in medical coding is important for two reasons. First, you need to know which codes to use for the services you provide. Second, you need to understand how the body works so that you can assign the correct codes when appropriate.

There are 11 major body systems: **integumentary, skeletal, muscular, nervous, endocrine, cardiovascular, lymphatic, immune system, respiratory system, digestive system, urinary system, and reproductive system.** Each of these systems has a variety of parts that work together to keep us alive and healthy.

For example, the respiratory system includes the nose and mouth as well as the lungs. When we breathe in air through our nose or mouth, it travels down our throat into our lungs. There it picks up oxygen from red blood cells before traveling back out through our nose or mouth again. This process allows us to get oxygen into our bloodstream so that we can stay alive!

Medical coders need a basic understanding of all 11 body systems in order to assign accurate codes for services provided by healthcare professionals. By learning about each individual body system, medical coders can more easily apply the correct code when necessary.

## Evaluation and Management Codes

Medical coding is a complex process that can be difficult to understand. One of the most important aspects of medical coding is understanding the evaluation and management codes. Evaluation and management codes are used to describe the type of visit that was performed by the doctor and to bill for those services. In this topic, we will explain what evaluation and management codes are, how they are used, and some common examples.

The first step in understanding evaluation and management codes is knowing what they are. Evaluation and management codes refer to a set of specific code numbers used to describe different types of doctor visits. These code numbers are assigned by the American Medical Association (AMA) CPT manual. The CPT manual contains all the current medical billing code numbers as well as descriptions for each code number.

**Evaluation and management codes can be used in two ways:**

- To report services provided during a visit.
- To report an office or other outpatient procedure performed during a visit.

**Services reported with an evaluation & management (E&M) code include:**
- ✓ history taking
- ✓ physical examination
- ✓ counseling/education

- ✓ coordination/direction
- ✓ tests interpretation

**Some common examples of when you would use an evaluation &management (E&M)code include:**

- ✓ New patient office visit
- ✓ Established patient office visit
- ✓ Consultation return visit
- ✓ Follow-up care after hospital discharge
- ✓ Emergency room encounter
- ✓ Home health care encounter
- ✓ Post-operative follow-up clinic appointment

CPT defines four levels of E&M service intensity which allow for more accurate reporting on physician time spent on various tasks:

**Level 1 -** typically 5 minutes or less face-to-face with the patient; minimal data gathering; minimal decision making.

**Level 2 -** typically more than 5 minutes but less than 10 minutes face-to-face with the patient; some data gathering; limited decision making.

**Level 3 -** typically more than 10 minutes but less than 30 minutes face-to - face with patients; extensive data gathering; Extensive decision making.

**Level 4 –** typically more than 30 minutes of face - to - face contact with patients; comprehensive history, extensive examination, extended counseling/education/coordination/direction.

To report services provided during a visit using an E&M Code: Report 99214 if it was billed separately from another service such as surgery.

## CHAPTER FIVE Understanding Commercial Health Insurance

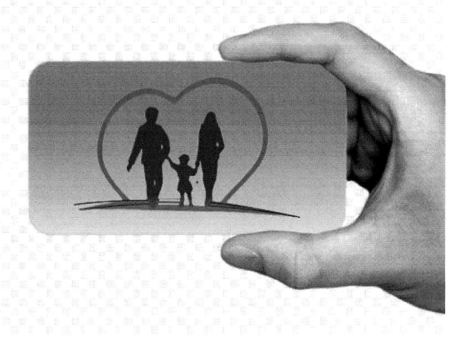

Having quality health insurance is important. But what do all of those terms mean? And how do you know which plan is right for your company? Here's a guide to understanding commercial health insurance:

Commercial health insurance is the most common type of health coverage in the United States. It's offered by employers and individual consumers, and it covers a wide range of services, from preventive care to hospitalization.

There are several different types of commercial health insurance plans, but they all share some common features:

✓ Coverage for preventive care services such as screenings and immunizations is free of charge.
✓ A deductible that must be paid before coverage begins.
✓ Coinsurance or copayments for most services.
✓ A maximum out-of-pocket amount that policyholders must pay each year.

**There are also several different types of commercial health insurance plans:**

**1) Health Maintenance Organizations (HMOs)** – An HMO is a type of managed care plan in which members receive their care from doctors who work for the HMO. Members usually have to choose a primary doctor who coordinates their care and refers them to specialists if needed.

**2) Preferred Provider Organizations (PPOs)** – A PPO is a type of managed care plan in which members can see any doctor they want, but they will generally pay less if they go to doctors who belong to the PPO network.

**3) Point-of-Service Plans (POS)** – Like PPOs, POS plans allow members to see any doctor they want; however, POS plans require members to get approval from their primary doctor before seeing a specialist.

**4) Exclusive Provider Organizations (EPOs)** – EPOs are like HMOs in that participants can only receive treatment from providers within the EPO network; however, there is no need for participants to designate one specific provider as their primary physician.

## The Right Way to Code Medicare Claims

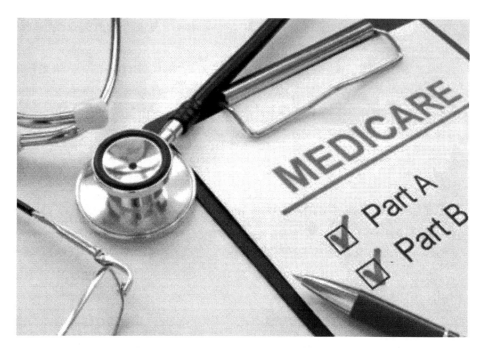

The billing portion of the process can seem complex for some healthcare providers, but the steps that you follow to complete a medical billing claim are very straightforward and should only take a few minutes of your time to complete.

**Step 1.** Review Your Medical Billing Information

The first step in the process is to gather and review the necessary information for processing a medical billing claim. For a standard claim, this information is a detailed summary of services provided and paid by the health insurance company (e.g. the hospital and physician). Depending on the type of insurance you carry, the insurance company may need additional information, such as authorization of the procedure and insurance forms, so this step may take more than a few minutes. If your medical bill is more complicated, you may have to dig through your insurance company's billing records, the medical chart, and medical records in order to complete your claim.

**Step 2.** File Your Medical Billing Claim

After you have compiled the required documentation to support your claim, it's time to submit it. This step can be quite straightforward, as many healthcare providers will have accounts with medical billing companies that will collect your information automatically. Regardless of the process that you use, keep in mind that many billing companies have a grace period of two business days to receive your claim. This two-day grace period is intended to allow billing companies to collect and pay bills before sending the total amount to your insurance company. Some insurance companies are strict about the number of days allowed for claim submission. Therefore, it is a good idea to check with your insurance company to make sure you can meet the deadline.

**Step 3.** Receive a Final Invoice

After submitting your claim, you will receive an invoice from the billing company that indicates the amount that your insurance company has paid. This amount is not the total amount that you will be reimbursed from your insurance company. Depending on your insurance policy, you may be able to apply the amount that you have been reimbursed toward future medical bills.

**Step 4.** Request Reimbursement from Your Insurance Company

After you receive your final invoice, it's time to send a letter or e-mail to your insurance company requesting reimbursement. Your insurance company will usually process the reimbursement within one or two business days. This reimbursement process varies depending on your insurance policy and type of service. For example, services like prescription drugs are generally covered by your insurance company before the final invoice is submitted, so your insurance company will likely cover those charges before you get reimbursed.

The amount that you are reimbursed can also vary depending on the type of service. This includes both the amount paid by your insurance company and the amount paid by your billing company. Some healthcare providers take advantage of billing companies by entering into contracts to set reimbursement amounts before the services are performed. For example, some hospitals have a separate agreement with a particular billing company that the hospital will charge for certain procedures.

These fees are collected in advance and a hospital can charge its patients the specified amount, regardless of the actual amount paid by the insurance company. These contracts can also take the place of a patient-physician relationship. In this case, there is no relationship between the hospital and the patient. The hospital collects a portion of the money paid by the insurance company to process the claim. If you are unsure about a specific agreement with a billing company, contact the billing company for more information.

**Step 5.** File a Refund Request

If you feel that you were over-paid by the insurance company, you can request a refund from your insurance company. This process may take a few days to complete, depending on the size of your insurance policy and the amount of the refund. Insurance companies typically require documentation to support the refund request. Your insurance company may also request some form of verification of the services that you received and the amount of the refund.

**Step 6.** Make a Record of the Claim

Finally, you need to make a note of the claim and keep the claim for some time. If your billing company does not require an electronic record of the claim, a paper copy of the bill and the patient statement is usually sufficient. Most insurance companies request electronic records of medical claims within a period of one to six months. These records allow the insurance company to monitor the types of procedures performed and the types of providers that are used in the treatment. It is also helpful to track the amount of time spent performing a procedure and the amount of reimbursement received. Some insurance companies have policies that require documentation of services performed, including an electronic record, in order to verify the services that are covered by the policy.

Completing a medical billing claim is a straightforward process that should only take a few minutes to complete. Many medical billing companies will take the work off of your hands and make it easy for you to submit a claim for reimbursement. If you have any questions about medical billing or insurance company requirements, feel free to contact your health insurance company for assistance.

## Understanding Medicaid Billing

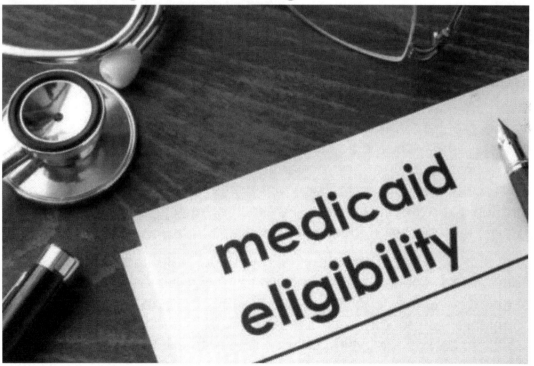

Medicaid is a program that offers health insurance for people who are poor and are on government assistance. In other words, it is the government's medical program for poor Americans. It is usually provided through hospitals, doctors, and pharmacies as a health insurance program. It is very similar to Medicare in concept. There is even a Medicare option. Medicaid is a state program, whereas Medicare is federally run.

Unlike private insurance plans, Medicaid does not require you to pay deductibles or a copayment first before it will pay for your care. Instead, Medicaid pays for all of your medical bills. In some states, it also covers your prescription drugs. It can, however, limit your coverage if you are enrolled in Medicare. In other words, if you are enrolled in Medicare, you cannot enroll in Medicaid. If you are uninsured or have health insurance through your employer, your health insurer will only cover your out-of-pocket costs.

**Why is the Medicaid program limited to Medicaid-eligible individuals only?**

It is a safety precaution. The Medicaid program only covers low-income people and no one else. It is not necessary for the survival of the program. There is no requirement that a person is poor in order to qualify for Medicaid. As a result, a person who can afford to pay a premium for an individual health insurance plan can afford to pay for his medical care. They just will have to pay out-of-pocket or through their employer. This may include a higher premium than a family insurance plan, depending on the policy.

The state Medicaid program is meant to help those who cannot afford their health insurance. Since it is limited to low-income people, there are fewer claims. This makes it easier for insurance companies to process claims because they have less medical billing and claims to review. With a larger group, there are more claims and more claims to review. With a smaller group, they have fewer claims to review, which is one of the reasons why their insurance premiums are lower.

**All You Need to Know About Patient Protection and Affordable Care Act (ACA)**

The Patient Protection and Affordable Care Act (ACA) also called ObamaCare, is a comprehensive health care reform law that was enacted in 2010. The ACA has made significant changes to the health care landscape in the United States, including provisions that expand access to coverage, improve quality of care, and reduce costs.

One of the most important aspects of the ACA is its expansion of Medicaid eligibility. As of January 1, 2014, all states were required to expand Medicaid eligibility to adults with incomes up to 138% of the federal poverty level. This expansion has helped millions of people gain access to affordable health coverage.

Another key provision of the ACA is its requirement that individuals have health insurance or pay a penalty. This "individual mandate" helps ensure that everyone has access to affordable coverage, regardless of their income or medical history. The individual mandate took effect on January 1, 2014 and applies to both uninsured individuals and those who purchase coverage through HealthCare.gov or a state-based exchange.

The ACA also includes provisions aimed at improving quality and reducing costs in our healthcare system. These include initiatives such as Accountable Care Organizations (ACOs) and bundled payments for episodes of care. ACOs are groups of doctors, hospitals, and other healthcare providers who come together voluntarily to provide coordinated high-quality care for their patients. Bundled payments are payments made by insurers for a package of services related to receiving treatment for an illness or injury. These initiatives aim to reward providers who deliver high-quality care while also reducing costs overall.

## Basic Certifications to Start a Promising Career as a Biller/Coder

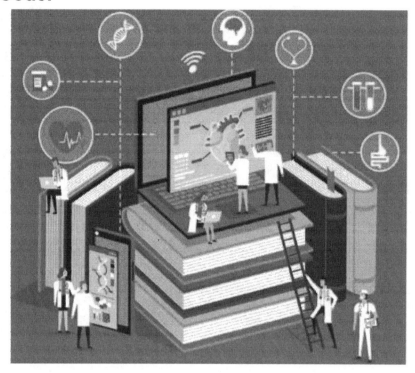

There are many basic certifications to start a promising career as a medical biller or coder. The most important factor is finding the right certification for your specific goals and interests.

The American Health Information Management Association (AHIMA) offers several certifications, such as the Certified Coding Associate (CCA) and Certified Coding Specialist (CCS). These credentials certify that you have the knowledge and skills to work with health information data and coding systems.

The National Healthcare Association (NHA) also offers certification options, such as their certified Billing & Coding Specialist program. This program helps students develop mastery of medical billing codes, claims processing, insurance reimbursement methods, and more.

No matter which certification you choose, make sure it is accredited by a reputable organization like AHIMA or NHA. This will ensure that your certificate has value in the workforce and meets industry standards.

# CHAPTER SIX A Review of the Exams

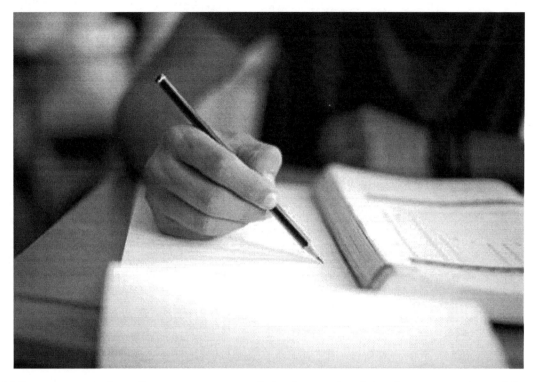

When preparing for any exam, it is important to have a plan. The same is true when studying for the Certified Medical Coder (CMC) or Certified Biller (CB) exams. Here are some general tips to help you get ready:

1. Start by reviewing the exam objectives. These outline what topics will be covered on the test. This will help you focus your studying and identify any areas that may need more attention.
2. Get familiar with the coding manuals. The CMC and CB exams both cover ICD-10-CM, HCPCS Level II, and AMA CPT codes, so it's important to know how to use

these resources correctly. Make sure you understand all the code changes that go into effect yearly on October 1st and January 1st.

3. Practice coding scenarios. There are many online practice quizzes available that can help you improve your coding skill set. Try answering questions from different types of charts – this will better prepare you for testing conditions!

4. Take practice tests. Similar to practicing coding scenarios, taking practice tests can help simulate test-day conditions and give you an idea of which topics may require more review time before taking the actual exam(s).

5. Finally, don't cram! It's important to allow yourself enough time for adequate preparation; trying to study everything overnight is not only ineffective but also counter-productive in most cases.

Following these tips should help prepare medical billers and coders for their certification exams!

## Getting Committed in Your Career Path as a Biller/Coder

If you're looking to get committed to your career path as a medical biller and coder, there are a few things you can do to set yourself up for success. Here are five tips that will help you stay on track:

I. Stay focused on your goals. It's easy to get sidetracked when you're working in the medical billing and coding field, but it's important to stay focused on your goals so you can continue progressing in your career. Make sure to set aside time each day to work on advancing your skills and learning new information.

II. Get involved with professional organizations. There are many professional organizations for medical billers and coders available online and offline, so be sure to get involved with one or more of them. This is a great way not only to learn more about the industry but also to make connections with other professionals who can help support and guide you along the way.

III. Network with others in the field. In addition to getting involved with professional organizations, networking is another great way to build relationships with others in the field of medical billing and coding. Attending conferences or meetups related specifically to his industry can provide opportunities for meeting other people who share your interests and ambitions – which could prove invaluable down the road!

IV. Use social media wisely. Social media platforms like LinkedIn offer great opportunities to connect with potential employers and colleagues from all over the world, so be sure to make use of these tools! Keep your profile updated and participate in relevant discussions that will help showcase y our expertise in this area.

V. Seek out, mentors. It never hurts to have someone experienced to guide you through the ups and downs of your career journey. Seek out mentors from within the industry who could provide valuable insights on how to achieve success in the medical billing and coding field.

## Signing Up and Getting Prepared for Study and Certification

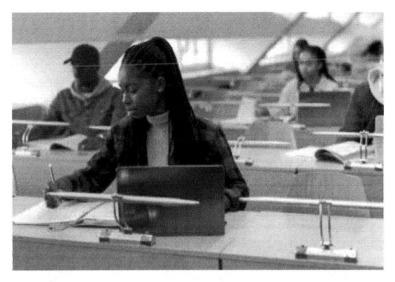

Choosing the right online medical billing and coding course is an important decision. There are many factors to consider when making your selection, such as cost, curriculum, and instructor quality.

The best way to find an online medical billing and coding course that meets your needs are to do some research. Start by reading reviews of different programs on websites like Indeed or Glassdoor. Once you've narrowed down your options, compare the courses side-by-side using a program comparison tool like Credible. When selecting an online medical billing and coding course, be sure to ask yourself the following questions:

## How much will it cost?

The price of a course can vary significantly depending on the school you choose. Make sure you're aware of all associated costs before enrolling (e.g., tuition, fees, textbooks). Some schools offer scholarships or financial aid opportunities which can help reduce the overall cost of attendance.

What's included in the curriculum? Curricula for online medical billing and coding courses vary widely from school to school. Make sure you know what topics will be covered so that you can be sure it matches your needs/interests. For example, if you're interested in pursuing a career as a coder rather than a biller then make sure that's reflected in the curriculum!

## Who are the instructors?

One of the most important factors when considering any educational program is who will be teaching it! Instructors should have experience in both teaching and work within the field they're instructing - this ensures that students receive both practical and theoretical instruction relevant to their chosen career path.

# CHAPTER SEVEN What a Perfect Billing Atmosphere Looks Like

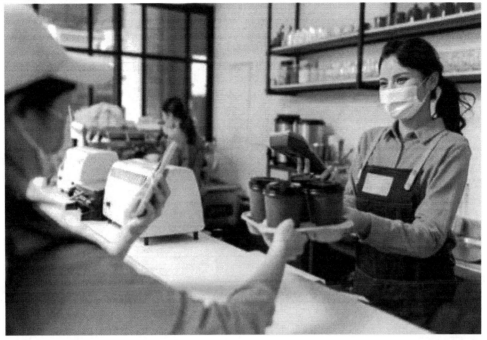

There is no one answer to this question since medical billing atmospheres can vary greatly from practice to practice. However, some general things would make any medical billing atmosphere perfect.

The first thing would be a friendly and helpful staff. The billers and coders should be knowledgeable and able to help patients with their questions. They should also be able to work efficiently so that bills are processed promptly.

Another important aspect of a perfect medical billing atmosphere is up-to-date technology. Billing software should be easy to use and accurate, as well as be updated regularly with the latest changes in insurance rules and regulations.

Finally, good communication is key in any office environment, especially so when it comes to medical billing. The staff needs to be able to effectively communicate with both the patients and the insurance companies in order to resolve any issues quickly and smoothly.

## Software Used for Medical Coding

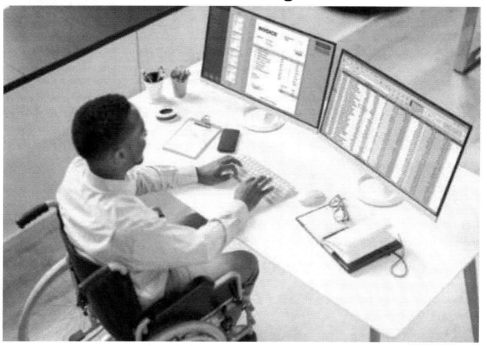

Medical coding and billing is a complex process that requires the use of specialized software. One of the most common pieces of software used in medical billing is an electronic health record (EHR) system. An EHR system allows healthcare providers to store patient data electronically, which can then be used for billing and other administrative purposes.

Another common piece of software used in medical coding and billing is a revenue cycle management (RCM) system. RCM systems are designed to help healthcare organizations manage their revenue by automating tasks such as claims submission, insurance verification, and payment processing.

Here are a few other lists of software:

**1. CPT Assistant:** This software is used to look up CPT codes. It includes information on code changes, guidelines, and more.

**2. ICD-10-CM:** This software is used to look up ICD-10 codes. It includes information on code changes, guidelines, and more.

**3. HCPCS Level II:** This software is used to look up HCPCS codes for outpatient services rendered by hospitals or other institutional providers (such as skilled nursing facilities). It includes information on code changes, guidelines, modifiers, etc.

**4. DRG Calculator:** This software helps identify diagnosis-related groups (DRGs) for hospital inpatient services.

**5. Medicare Fee Schedules:** This software provides fee schedule data for physicians' services under the Medicare program.

## Understanding Medical Billing Contracts

Medical billing contracts are a form of healthcare insurance that physicians and practices can use to contract with insurers or health plans. Some doctors, especially those who do not have a strong practice infrastructure, contract with insurance plans or plans directly for their medical billing services. These physicians may also work with a medical billing consultant. Medical billing services that are contracted by a physician are generally an add-on to the physician's overall payment, although some physicians contract for additional cash.

For instance, a physician may be paid a flat fee for a number of services performed during the month; however, this fee is likely to be less than what the physician could be paid if the services were billed directly. A physician who contracts for his or her medical billing services, or some of them, will have less overhead expenses and be able to spend more time working with patients. However, the most important consideration for a physician who uses a medical billing consultant is that it costs more upfront to contract a medical billing consultant than to perform medical billing services on an ongoing basis.

When a physician uses a medical billing consultant, he or she must pay this cost in addition to what he or she normally charges. This will depend on the services contracted for, the experience of the medical billing consultant, and the physician's financial health. If a physician has any doubt that he or she can handle medical billing, he or she should consider using a medical billing consultant, as he or she will most likely save more money on the actual medical billing procedures.

There are many types of medical billing and reimbursement systems that a medical billing consultant can work with. The most common types of systems include:

- ✓ The American Medical Association's (AMA)
- ✓ Current Procedural Terminology (CPT) system
- ✓ The Healthcare Finance Corporation's Electronic Health Record (EHR) system
- ✓ The Medical Practice Systems (MPS) system
- ✓ The OpenEMR system

Some other medical billing consultants work with practice management systems that combine all of the medical billing information into one database system. These systems are usually integrated with practice management systems. The contracts for medical billing services will usually include an initial fee for a set time. This fee will cover most or all the medical billing and reimbursement services to be provided. However, some medical billing contracts for medical billing services allow a physician to renew their contract for an additional period at a discount. If you have any questions about medical billing contracts, ask your consultant for details.

## Types of Medical Billing Services Contract

There are many types of medical billing services contracts for physicians to choose from. The first is a medical billing and reimbursement agreement that is usually with an insurance company or third-party payer. This is also known as a medical billing contract. This is where the physician works directly with the third-party payer to handle all medical billing and payments for his or her office. However, some insurance plans prefer to handle the medical billing in-house and the physician is paid a set flat fee for this service.

The second type of medical billing service is one where a medical billing consultant is hired by a practice. This is more of a service contract, where a doctor may use a medical billing consultant for certain services as needed. The services contracted for will depend on the kind of medical billing system used by the practice.

The third type of medical billing service is one where the medical billing consultant is hired by a doctor and the physician also contracts for the medical billing consultant's services for a while. This is one of the most common types of medical billing service contracts for physicians.

## Referrals and Prior Authorization in Medical Billing

As a medical biller, it is important to understand the referral and prior authorization process. A referral is when a doctor refers a patient to another doctor or specialist for treatment. The referral may be for an evaluation or treatment. Prior authorization is when insurance approves certain treatments before they are given to the patient.

There are several reasons why doctors may refer patients to other doctors or specialists. One reason may be that the doctor does not have the necessary expertise to treat the condition. Another reason may be because of geographical limitations, such as if there are no specialists in the area who can treat the condition. Sometimes referrals are made because of insurance limitations, such as when a procedure is not covered by insurance or there is a limit on how many times it can be done in a year.

The referral and prior authorization process begin with the doctor who referred the patient and sending information about the patient to another doctor or specialist. This information usually includes:

✓ The name and contact information of both doctors
✓ The diagnosis
✓ Any tests that have been done
✓ A list of medications that have been prescribed

Once this information has been sent, it is up to both doctors involved in treating the patient to work out any arrangements for care between themselves. This includes deciding which hospital the patient will go to between them and setting up appointments for evaluations or treatments. If either doctor needs approval from insurance before providing care, then prior authorization will need to be processed.

# CHAPTER EIGHT Claim Tracking in Medical Billing

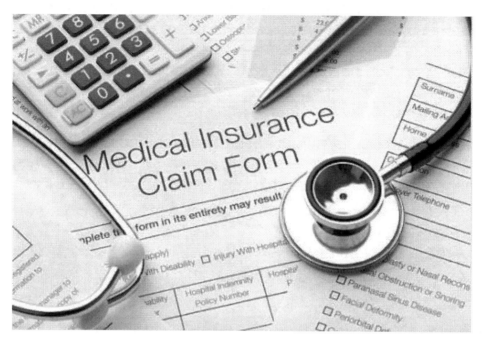

Medical billing can be a complex and confusing process. This guide will help you understand how to track medical claims and ensure that you are being properly reimbursed for the services you provide.

The first step in tracking medical claims is understanding the insurance claim process. There are three main players in this process: the provider, the payer, and the patient. The provider is responsible for delivering healthcare services, the payer is responsible for reimbursing providers for those services, and the patient is responsible for paying any out-of-pocket costs.

The second step in tracking medical claims is understanding your contract with each of your payers. This contract will outline what services are covered by that particular payer, as well as what reimbursement rates you can expect. It's important to review this information regularly so that you can be sure that you're being fairly compensated for your services.

The third step in tracking medical claims is keeping track of all of your billing paperwork. This includes both electronic and paper invoices/statements, as well as any accompanying documentation such as EOBs (explanation of benefits) or remittance advice (RA). You'll need to keep this information organized so that it's easy to find when needed - especially if there are any questions or disputes about a particular claim later on down the line.

## Procedures for Starting an Appeal in Medical Billing

If you've received a medical bill that you feel is unfair or too high, don't panic. You may be able to appeal the bill and get it lowered. Here are the steps to take:

➢ Review your medical bill and make sure all the services listed were provided to you. If something doesn't seem right, contact your healthcare provider immediately.
➢ Compare your medical bill with what Medicare would have paid for the same services (you can find this information on medicare.gov). If your provider charged more than Medicare would have, you may be able to appeal the charge as being unfair or unreasonable.
➢ Gather evidence to support your appeal, such as doctor notes or receipts for medications/supplies purchased outside of the hospital setting.
➢ Complete an Appeal Form (you can find this on medicareadvocacy.org) and send it along with all of your supporting documentation to your health insurance company.
➢ Wait for a response from your health insurance company – they should let you know whether they accept or deny your appeal within 60 days.

- ➤ If denied, go through step two again and gather even more evidence in support of your claim.
- ➤ Finally, if still denied after exhausting all appeals available through your health insurance company, consider filing a complaint with the Centers for Medicare & Medicaid Services (CMS).

## What are CPT Codes?

CPT codes are a set of numbers and letters that represent medical procedures and services. They are used by doctors, insurance companies, and other healthcare providers to bill for services rendered. The use of CPT codes allows for uniformity in the billing process across all healthcare settings.

There are thousands of CPT codes, which can be confusing to understand. However, with a little bit of knowledge, it is possible to decode these important numbers. In this guide, we will provide an overview of what CPT codes are and how they work, as well as some tips on how to find the right code for a specific procedure or service.

CPT stands for Current Procedural Terminology. It is a set of standard medical billing codes developed by the American Medical Association (AMA). These numeric and alphanumeric identifiers describe medical procedures and services so that they may be billed uniformly between providers nationwide. There are currently over 10,000 different codes of the three categories of CPT codes in use. Each code has its description, definition, usage notes, modifiers, etc. The AMA updates the coding system annually with new procedures and changes to existing ones.

## How do I find the right code?

Figuring out which CPT code applies to a particular procedure or service can be tricky - there is no one-size-fits-all answer! However, some general tips can help make finding the right code easier:

**1) Start with what you know:** Begin by looking up common procedures in your field using online resources such as UpToDate or PubMed Clinical Queries.

**2) Use official resources:** When you're not sure about which code applies or need clarification on usage rules/notes etc., consult official sources such as CMS's Medicare Fee Schedule database

**3) Ask your colleagues:** Other coders or clinicians who have experience with specific procedures may also be able to offer guidance.

**4) Check CCI edits:** If you're unsure whether two particular codes can safely be billed together (for example because they might result in incorrect reimbursement), check out CCI edits via Medlearn Matters.

**5) Use code lookup tools:** A variety of online tools exist specifically designed to help users locate appropriate codes given their clinical scenario - one popular option is ICD10 lookup from HCPCS Level II.

## How are CPT Codes Assigned?

CPT codes are the numerical codes that represent medical, surgical, and diagnostic services. They are used to bill insurance companies for services rendered by healthcare providers. The CPT code assignment process can be confusing for those who are not familiar with it. This guide will help you understand how CPT codes are assigned so that you can be better informed when making decisions about your healthcare.

CPT coding is a complex process that involves many different factors. The following is a brief overview of the three main methods used to assign CPT codes:

**1) Clinical Documentation:** Healthcare providers use clinical documentation to provide an accurate description of the service they have provided to their patients. This documentation is then used to determine which CPT code should be assigned to the service in question.

**2) National Correct Coding Initiative (NCCI):** The NCCI edits identify specific services that should not be billed together because they may result in an incorrect claim being processed by insurance companies.

**3) Relative Value Units (RVUs):** RVUs are determined by Medicare and reflect the relative value of each procedure based on time, intensity, skill level, and other resources required.

The first step in assigning a CPT code is determining which category the service falls into. There are five categories: Evaluation & Management Services;

- ➤ Medical Services;
- ➤ Surgical Services;
- ➤ Radiology Services;
- ➤ Laboratory & Pathology Services.

Once you have determined which category your service falls in, you can then begin looking at specific procedures within that category.

**Evaluation & Management Procedures:** These procedures include office visits, consultations, telephone calls, etc., and usually involve some type of assessment or evaluation of a patient's condition.

**Medical Procedures:** These procedures typically involve treatment or intervention for a particular condition or illness.

**Surgical Procedures:** These procedures involve actual surgery performed on a patient.

**Radiology Procedures:** These procedures include X-rays, MRIs, CT scans, etc., as well as radiation therapy.

**Laboratory & Pathology Procedures:** These procedures include tests such as blood work or biopsies.

## Using Modifiers in Medical Billing/Coding

One of the most confusing aspects of medical billing and coding is modifiers. Modifiers are used to indicate specific details about a procedure or service, and they can affect how much you're billed for that procedure or service.

In this detailed guide to modifiers in medical billing and coding, we'll explain what modifiers are, how they're used, and the different types of modifiers. We'll also provide some examples to help you better understand how these codes work. Let's get started!

## What are modifiers?

Modifiers are codes that indicate specific details about a procedure or service. They may be used to indicate changes made during surgery, such as adding incision; changes in the way a service was provided; or unusual circumstances surrounding a procedure or service.

Modifiers can also be used to report on services rendered by other providers (such as anesthesiologists) who were not involved in providing care for the patient on the date of service.

## How are modifiers used?

There are two ways that modifiers can be used: modifier -51 (indicating surgical assistant) and modifier -52 (indicating surgical assistant when no operative report was available). In addition, there are three ways that modifier -59 may be appended:

1) When multiple procedures were performed on one day but only one E/M code is reported;

2) When two procedures were done at different times on the same day with the same documentation;

3) When there is more than one encounter during which services were provided but only one E/M code was reported.

What types of modifier codes are there? There are five types of modifier codes: global period, add-on, reporting, bilateral/unilateral, and professional component.

**Global Period:** A global period indicates how long after surgery your surgeon will bill for his/her services.

**Add-on:** An add-on code indicates additional work that was done above and beyond what was originally billed. It could include time spent performing an extra test or ordering supplies not related to the original diagnosis.

**Reporting:** A reporting code tells us which type of information is being conveyed by the modifier – usually whether it's related to an operative report (OR), anesthesia report (ANES), pathology & laboratory report (PATH), radiology report (RADIOL), or another type of medical report.

**Bilateral/Unilateral:** A bilateral modifier code is used in medical billing to indicate that a service was provided on both sides of the body. For example, if you provide physical therapy services to a patient on both the left and right sides of their body, you would use the bilateral modifier code (CPT 97001). This would tell the insurance company that they should pay for two sessions of physical therapy, rather than just one.

A unilateral modifier code is used in medical billing to indicate that a service was provided on only one side of the body. For example, if you provide physical therapy services to a patient on only their left side, you would use the unilateral modifier code (CPT 97002). This would tell the insurance company that they should pay for one session of physical therapy, rather than two.

Professional component: In the medical billing profession, a professional component modifier code is used to indicate that a service was provided by a qualified professional. This modifier is used in conjunction with other codes to indicate the level of service provided. For example, if you were to see a chiropractor for treatment, you would use the code CPT 98940 which indicates that treatment was performed by a chiropractor. If you were to see a physical therapist instead, you would use CPT 97001 which indicates that treatment was performed by a physical therapist. The use of this modifier allows insurers and healthcare providers to more accurately track services provided by qualified professionals.

## Understanding Edits in Medical Billing

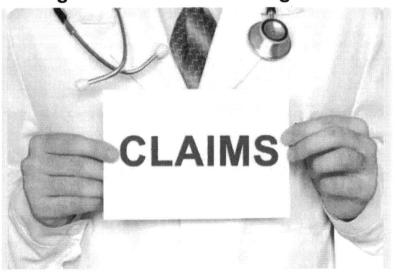

Edits are an important part of the medical billing process. They ensure that claims are accurate and processed properly. This detailed guide will help you understand what claim edits are, how they're applied, and how to appeal them if necessary.

## What is a claim edit?

A claim edit is an adjustment to a medical bill that is made by the insurance company. The purpose of these edits is to ensure that the claims being submitted are accurate and meet all the insurance company's requirements. There are many different types of claim edits, and each one can have a significant impact on your bottom line.

How are claim edits applied?

The way in which claim edits are applied varies depending on the type of edit involved. Generally speaking, however, there are two main methods:

Claim editing software compares each line item on your bill against specific criteria set by the insurer. If something doesn't match up - such as an incorrect procedure code or missing information then it will be flagged as an error and may be subject to adjustment.

A claims adjuster reviews all the bills submitted for a given patient/claims file and makes manual adjustments as needed based on their judgment about what's appropriate under those circumstances.

# CHAPTER NINE All You Need to Know About Clearinghouse inMedical Claims

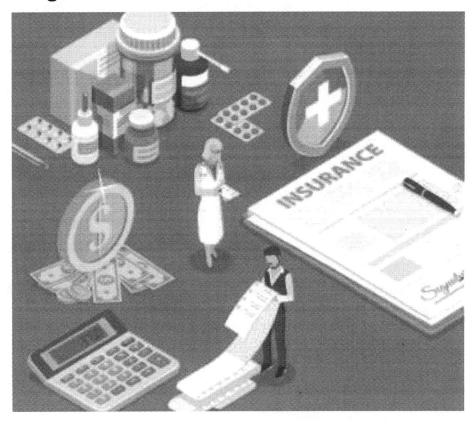

You may have heard the term clearinghouse mentioned, but not be sure what it means. A clearinghouse is a company that helps insurance companies and healthcare providers exchange information related to medical claims. Clearinghouses are often used to process and manage electronic health care transactions.

There are many benefits of using a clearinghouse for your practice. They can help you save time and money by reducing claim rejections, improving data accuracy, and helping you meet compliance regulations.

If you're considering using a clearinghouse for your practice, here's what you need to know:

- ➤ Clearinghouses typically charge a fee for their services
- ➤ They can help improve data accuracy by validating patient information against insurance company databases
- ➤ They can also help reduce claim rejections caused by incorrect or incomplete information
- ➤ Some clearinghouses offer additional services such as eligibility verification and prior authorization assistance.

## Fundamentals of Medical Reimbursement and Coding

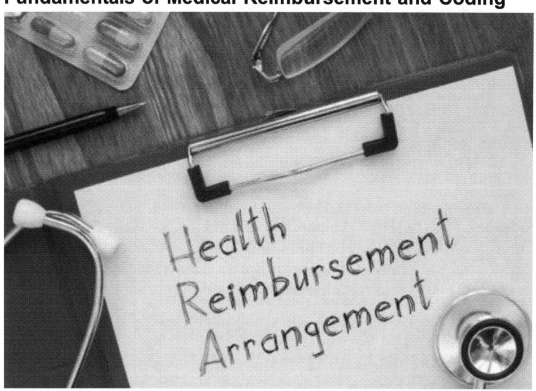

Medical reimbursement and coding are critical parts of the healthcare industry. It involves the classification of medical services and procedures according to specific codes that are used to bill patients, insurance companies, and other third-party payers. The goal of medical reimbursement and coding is to ensure that everyone involved in the billing process is accurately billed for the services they provided.

There are two main types of medical coding: diagnosis coding and procedure coding. Diagnosis codes identify specific diseases or conditions, while procedure codes identify the type of service or treatment that was provided. There are also several levels of specificity within each type of code.

For example, there are general diagnosis codes as well as more specific diagnosis codes for different types of cancer, heart disease, etc. Similarly, there are general procedure codes as well as more specific procedure codes for things like surgery, radiology procedures, etc.

The use of medical reimbursement and coding standards helps ensure uniformity in how services are billed across different providers and locations. This not only simplifies billing but also makes it easier to track payments made by insurance companies and other third-party payers. In addition, these standards help protect patients from being overcharged for services rendered.

## Understanding Ambulance Transportation Billing

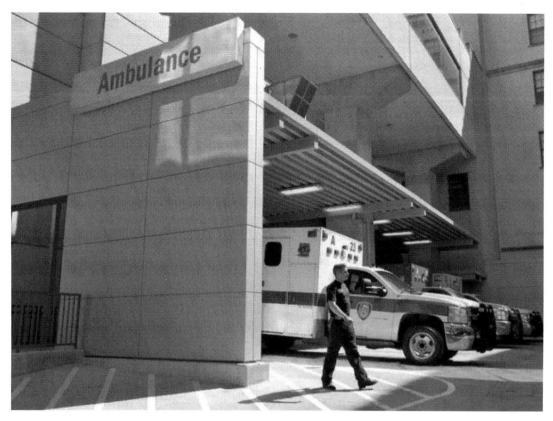

Ambulance transportation billing in healthcare can be confusing. It is important to understand the basics of how ambulance transportation billing works in order to make sure you are being billed correctly and know what your responsibility is when it comes to paying for ambulance services.

The first thing to understand is that there are two types of ambulance transport: emergency and non-emergency. Emergency transport is provided when a patient's life or health is in danger, while non-emergency transport typically refers to transports that are not considered emergencies, such as transports for routine dialysis appointments or cancer treatments.

Emergency transport services are typically covered by insurance, while non-emergency transports may not be covered depending on your plan. It's important to check with your insurance company before you need an ambulance ride so you know what your coverage entails. In most cases, though, if you do need an ambulance for a non-emergency ride, you will be responsible for paying the bill yourself.

The cost of an ambulance ride varies depending on the type of service and where it takes place. Generally speaking, emergency rides cost more than non-emergencies because they involve additional resources like paramedics and medical equipment. However, prices can vary widely based on location so it's best to contact your local EMS agency directly if you have any specific questions about costs involved with using their services.

Ambulance bills can be complicated, so it's important to familiarize yourself with all the charges involved in order to ensure that they are billed correctly. If there are any discrepancies on the bill, contact your insurance company immediately so that they can investigate further.

## Understanding Coding and Claim Denials

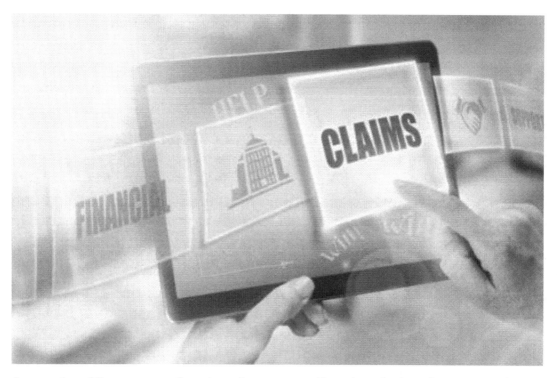

As a healthcare professional, you understand the importance of coding and claim denials. However, do you know how to read and understand coding? In order to ensure that your practice is running smoothly and efficiently, it's important to be well-versed in both.

As you know, coding is the process of transforming patient information into universal medical codes that can be used for billing and insurance purposes. These codes are used to track patient diagnoses, procedures performed, medications given, etc. Claim denials occur when an insurer denies a claim for payment because it doesn't meet their specific criteria or because there is an error on the part of the provider or insurer.

While both coding and claim denials may seem daunting at first glance, they are quite easy to understand with a little bit of guidance. In this topic, we will provide a detailed guide on how to read and interpret coding as well as what you can do if your claims are denied. Let's get started!

Before we dive into decoding specific medical codes, let's take a quick look at how coding works in general:

- ❖ The coder takes information from the patient's chart including symptoms, diagnosis codes (ICD-10), procedures performed (CPT), etc., and translates them into standard code numbers.
- ❖ This coded data is then submitted along with charges for services rendered.
- ❖ If there are any errors on the submission (e.g., incorrect code numbers or charges), these will be flagged by insurers during the pre-payment review.
- ❖ If everything looks good after the pre-payment review, the claim will go through and payment will be issued.
- ❖ If there are any issues after the pre-payment review, the insurer may deny the entire claim or just certain portions depending on what was found wrong.

Now that you have an overview of how coding works let's move on to decoding those pesky medical codes!

Decoding CPT Codes can be more complicated because they often include modifiers, which change or add details about how a procedure was performed. For example, Here's an excerpt from CPT Code 99214: "Extended evaluation and management service; moderate complexity," this code indicates that it's for an extended evaluation and management service provided at a moderate level of complexity. To find out what exactly constitutes "moderate complexity," you would need to refer to the modifier definitions section of the coder's manual.

So now that you understand how decoding works, here are some tips for making sense of your medical bills:

1) Make sure that you identify the correct code set before trying to decode any information.

2) When in doubt, consult with either your doctor or coder friend! They will likely have access to resources like online coding manuals.

## Remittance Advice in Billing Process

When it comes to understanding medical billing, one of the most important aspects is understanding remittance advice. This document accompanies a bill and outlines what was billed, what insurance paid, and what the patient owes. It can be confusing to decipher at first, but with a little bit of knowledge, it's easy to understand the basics.

The first section of remittance advice will list all the services that were billed for the visit. Each service will have its line item with information on how much was charged, how much insurance was paid, and how much is left for the patient to pay.

Next is an explanation of why certain charges were not paid by insurance. This section can be confusing because there are often codes associated with each reason. However, most patients don't need to worry about decoding these codes - they just need to know which ones indicate that their insurer didn't cover a particular service or charge.

Finally, any payments made by both the insurer and patient will be listed here along with their respective totals. This section can help patients keep track of exactly how much money they still owe after insurance has covered its portion.

# CHAPTER TEN Thorough Guide for Settling Disputes and MakingAppeals

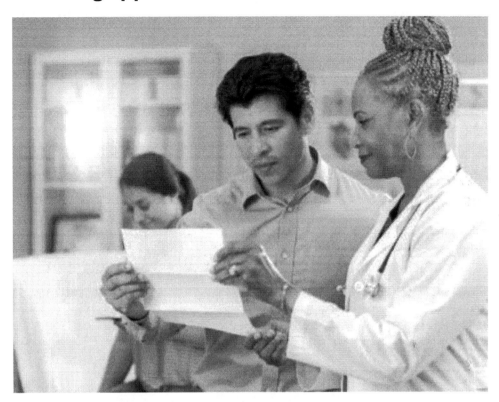

Medical billing disputes and the appeal process are the primary means that a healthcare provider uses to address an error in payment, a medical bill, or a denial of insurance coverage. The primary goal of the appeal is to achieve the highest reimbursement amount for the treatment of the patient. There are many factors that will affect your medical billing dispute and appeal. The following are some of the most common factors and issues that need to be considered.

The appeal process is not a one-time process. It will require the help of someone who understands the different insurance and payment options. They will be able to help you with the insurance, payer, and health care system. As a medical professional you should be more than willing to learn about this process. You should be able to teach your office staff about this process so they can handle this in the future.

Most disputes or disputes between insurance companies will be settled outside the court system. Most of these disputes will be resolved through the different payers and insurance companies involved. They will agree on a settlement amount for the number of services provided. Then they will be able to resolve any differences in the medical billing and appeal processes. The other option is to have your case go before a judge. The judge will look at the evidence to see if you are entitled to the reimbursement amount and to be granted. He or she will make a decision on whether to approve or deny your request for reimbursement.

## How will I appeal an insurance decision that does not approve my request for reimbursement?

You will have the choice of appealing the decision or agreeing with the decision. This is a legal right that is given to you as a medical provider. If you agree with the insurance company's decision then you will have to pay the amount of the bill. If you disagree with the insurance company then you have a few options available to you. You can appeal the decision in court. If this is a dispute between an insurance company and a medical provider, you can file your case in the courts. The decision can then be reviewed by a judge. If you are able to show that the insurance company incorrectly processed your bill and that you are entitled to the funds, then the judge will likely order the insurance company to reimburse you.

You can also accept a payment plan that allows you to receive the payments that you are owed. The best way to accept this type of payment is by signing up for a third-party online platform. They have a network of providers and providers that are willing to take on the responsibility of making payments to providers every month. The best option is the Patient Advocate Network (PAN). This service allows you to accept payments from health insurance companies, Medicare, Medicaid, and Private Pay, and they will send the reimbursement directly to you in your preferred form of payment. You can choose from four options. You can receive an ACH payment, EFT payment, paper check, or credit card payment.

## What happens if the amount of the payment I am asking for is less than the amount I am billed?

If you are entitled to the total amount that is being billed then the insurance company is required to pay you the full amount. If you are asking for a larger amount than the insurance company has paid you in the past, they may be hesitant to pay more money for the same service. They will usually offer you a settlement amount to avoid having to go through the appeal process. This is a very common approach by health care companies and insurance companies when they have made an error in payment for a medical provider. They will send you a payment that is higher than the amount that you are requesting. They may ask you to sign a release agreement. This is a document that will release the insurance company from any liability if any disputes arise after the settlement. They will be able to deny any responsibility for the case if you sign this.

## What will happen if I lose the medical billing dispute?

Your case may end up before a judge or it may be resolved without a judge. If your case is resolved without a judge, it will go before a reviewer. The reviewer will look at all the evidence that was presented to them by both parties and they will decide what will be awarded to you. The reviewer may award more or less than the original amount that was billed to you by the insurance company or hospital. If you choose to go through the judicial system, the judge will review all the evidence presented to him or her. They will look at everything that has been requested for reimbursement. They will look at all the documentation that has been requested to see if you are entitled to the money. If you do not receive the amount that was agreed upon by the insurance company, the judge will make a ruling to decide the amount that you will receive. If you find that the judge is unable to decide the case in your favor, then you can appeal to the appellate court. If you are not able to agree with the decision that was reached by the judge then you can choose to have the judge review the evidence.

## What happens if my claim was denied and I cannot agree with the judge's ruling?

If your appeal is approved then the amount will be forwarded to the insurance company or payer in question. If you disagree with the ruling then you can file an appeal. The insurance company or payer will be notified and they can either agree with your request or they can ask the court to reconsider. The court will then decide if the amount was correct or not. If it was not then they can give you the amount that they feel is correct or they can award you with the amount that was originally sent to you by the insurance company. If you disagree with the court ruling, you may want to file an appeal. In this case, you can choose to file the appeal directly with the appellate court. This is an appeal that will go before a higher court that will look at the evidence that was presented and the reasoning behind the court's decision.

## What happens if my appeal is denied by the appellate court?

If your appeal is denied then you can request a reconsideration. You can file this request in a different county than the county in that your appeal was filed. In order to do this, you will need to contact the appellate court in the county that you would like to appeal. The court will decide if the evidence presented in the appeal was sufficient to justify reconsideration. If they are not, then they will deny your request. If your appeal is denied again then you can file a request for a rehearing. Your request will be sent to the appellate court that originally denied your appeal. This is your final chance to have your appeal approved. You can choose to have a lawyer represent you, but you will need to pay for the services of your attorney. This will include having an initial consultation, filing the request for a rehearing, and any appeals that need to be filed after that.

## Understanding ICD Codes

The International Classification of Diseases (ICD) is the standard set of codes that are used to classify various illnesses and diseases. There are some other classification systems, however, the ICD is the most accepted system. The ICD codes are used by doctors, and health professionals to classify the visit and the patient's condition. These are also used by the government and private insurance companies to report on the details of the visits to the hospitals, and health facilities. ICD codes are classified into different categories and sub-categories. The codes are related to the diagnosis and type of services performed.

The codes are provided by the World Health Organization (WHO) and are also divided based on the countries. The first digit indicates the disease code, while the remaining digits relate to the type of ICD code. For example, when a patient visits a doctor, the doctor would record the reason for the visit. This is used to classify the illness, and a specific code is assigned. The code is assigned by the physician who is treating the patient. The next step is to check the database and see the ICD code related to the illness. The codes are classified based on the body systems. The body systems such as the respiratory system, digestive system, musculoskeletal system, etc.

## The Role of Payers in the Medical Billing Process

The role of payers in a medical billing process is critical. They are responsible for ensuring that claims are filed accurately and paid on time. In addition, they work with providers to help ensure that patients receive the most appropriate care.

There are several types of payers, including insurance companies, government programs, and self-pay patients. Each one has its own set of rules and regulations that must be followed when filing claims.

Insurance companies are the primary payers for medical bills, they contract with healthcare providers to provide coverage for their members. In order to file a claim with an insurance company, you will need the member's ID number and policy information.

Government programs include Medicare and Medicaid. These programs are funded by taxpayers and provide health coverage for seniors, disabled individuals, and low-income families respectively Medicare is a federally funded program while Medicaid is a state-funded program. However, each state sets its eligibility requirements. For example, California has different eligibility requirements than Texas. To file a claim with Medicare or Medicaid, you will need the beneficiary's social security number or Medicaid ID number.

Self-pay patients account for about 10% of all healthcare payments; this can be individuals who do not have insurance or those who have exhausted their benefits Most hospitals offer financial assistance options such as payment plans or discounts. For self-pay patients, it is important to contact the hospital billing office directly to establish payment arrangements.

In order to ensure accurate reimbursement, it is important to understand how each type of payer processes claims. The role of payers in medical billing can seem daunting but by understanding their guidelines it becomes much easier.

## Maximizing Insurance Plans in Medical Billing

Maximizing your insurance plan is key to minimizing your medical billing expenses. In order to do this, you need to be familiar with the different aspects of your insurance coverage.

First, you should understand the basics of how health insurance plans work. Most plans are either indemnity or managed care plans. An indemnity plan allows you freedom of choice in selecting a doctor and usually has a higher premium. A managed care plan typically restricts you to a specific network of doctors but may have lower premiums and co-pays.

It is important to know which type of plan you have so that you can take advantage of its benefits. For example, an indemnity plan might cover 100% after a deductible is met for out-of-network services, while a managed care plan would only cover 50%.

Additionally, it's important to read through your policy carefully and understand the terms and conditions associated with each benefit offered by your insurer. This will help ensure that when services are provided, they are billed correctly and covered by your insurance company according. To maximize these benefits make sure service codes matchup between what's being billed by healthcare providers and the description of the service listed on the insurance company's website as well as any Explanation Of Benefits (EOB) statements received after treatment.

# CHAPTER ELEVEN Working with Medicare Contractors

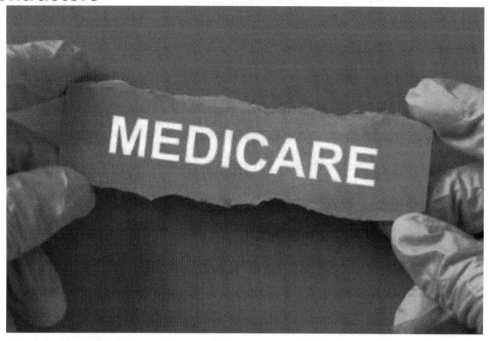

As a medical biller, you will likely need to work with Medicare administrative contractors (MACs) to process and submit claims on behalf of your healthcare organization. This detailed guide will provide an overview of the role of MACs in the Medicare program, as well as tips on how to work effectively with them.

## What are Medicare administrative contractors?

Medicare administrative contractors are private companies that have been contracted by the Centers for Medicare & Medicaid Services (CMS) to administer various aspects of the Medicare program. There are 10 regional MACs in total, each responsible for a specific geographic area.

The duties of MACs include processing and paying claims, auditing provider billing practices, and responding to customer inquiries.

## How do I work with a MAC?

There is no one-size-fits-all answer when it comes to working with a MAC – it can vary depending on which contractor you're dealing with and what services they offer. However, some general tips can help make the process smoother:

- ❖ Be familiar with your local MAC's policies and procedures.
- ❖ Make sure all claim information is complete and accurate.
- ❖ Submit claims promptly – preferably within 30 days of the service date.
- ❖ Follow up on rejected or denied claims promptly.
- ❖ Keep good records relating to all interactions with your local MAC.

## Understanding Medicare Advantage Plans

Medicare Advantage Plans are a type of health insurance plan offered by private companies that contract with Medicare to provide benefits. These plans include all the benefits of Original Medicare (Part A and Part B), plus additional services like vision, dental, and hearing care.

There are many different types of Medicare Advantage Plans available, so it's important to understand which one is right for you. The most common types are:

**HMO** – An HMO plan requires you to use doctors, hospitals, and other healthcare providers in the plan's network. If you go outside the network for care, you may have to pay more out-of-pocket.

**PPO** – A PPO plan allows you to use doctors and hospitals outside of the plan's network but usually at a higher cost.

**POS** – A POS plan is similar to an HMO but gives you some flexibility in using out-of-network providers. You may have to pay more out-of-pocket if you do this than if you use in-network providers though.

**SNP** – A Special Needs Plan is designed specifically for people who have certain chronic conditions or meet certain eligibility criteria like being over 65 or disabled.

## Improving the Billing Experience for Your Patients

As a healthcare provider, you're likely always looking for ways to improve the billing experience for your patients. After all, this is an important part of their overall experience with your practice.

Fortunately, there are a number of things you can do to make the billing process smoother and easier for your patients. Here's a detailed guide on how to improve the billing experience for your patients:

1) Make sure that you have clear and concise billing information available on your website. This should include an overview of what to expect from the billing process, as well as contact information if patients have any questions or concerns.

2) Try to keep patient bills organized and easy to read. Use clear headings and formatting so that patients can quickly understand what they're being charged for.

3) Be proactive in communicating with patients about their bills. Let them know when charges have been processed and provide updates if there are any changes or discrepancies with their billings.

4) Offer payment options that are convenient for your patients. This could include online payments, automatic withdrawals from bank accounts, or even in-person payments at local pharmacies or grocery stores.

5) Respond promptly to any inquiries from Patients regarding their bills. Address any concerns they may have and provide additional clarification if needed.

## Understanding Patient Confidentiality in Medical Billing and Coding

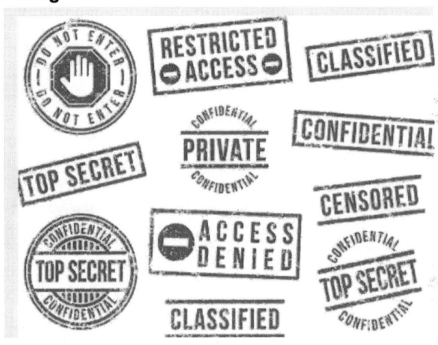

As a medical billing and coding professional, your priority is to secure patient trust. You can earn this trust, however, only when you demonstrate your confidentiality at the highest level. The best way to maintain the trust of your patients is to communicate directly with them whenever possible and to always keep their information confidential.

In the practice of medical billing and coding, confidentiality refers to the principle that, whenever possible, patient information must be kept secure and must not be disclosed or transmitted in ways that could harm the patient's interest. Medical professionals have to be cognizant of the confidential nature of patient information and protect it.

Medical billing and coding records are some of the most important documents we maintain in our practices. If you have any information pertaining to your patient (such as medical history, medical bills, laboratory results, insurance cards, test results, and much more), it is crucial to take the necessary steps to protect it. Patients have an expectation of the utmost confidentiality in medical care. To fulfill that obligation, billing and coding professionals must exercise both physical and psychological barriers against the leakage of sensitive patient information.

This obligation has recently become particularly important because of the growing concern about security breaches, including computer hacks, medical record leaks, and unencrypted personal information. Healthcare providers have a legal duty to protect the privacy and confidentiality of a patient's medical records. They need to realize that this obligation extends to the information they provide about their patients to insurance companies, governmental agencies, and law enforcement officials.

This confidentiality is very important to the patient. Not only do patients have a legitimate expectation that their confidential medical information will be kept private and secure, it also puts the provider at a disadvantage in negotiating higher fees. A provider may receive a penalty from a patient's insurance company for failing to treat his or her medical condition as promised. It is to a patient's advantage to have a confidential and secure relationship with a medical provider. Patients have a right to expect that their medical information will be kept private and secure.

## The Best Way to Collect Patient Payments in Medical Billing and Coding

Medical billing professionals are responsible for ensuring that patient payments are collected in a timely and efficient manner. In order to do so, it is important to understand the best tips for collecting payments from patients.

1. Make sure that your billing procedures are clear and easy to understand. Patients should know what is expected of them when it comes to paying their bills.

2. Send out invoices promptly and ensure that they are accurate. If there are any questions or discrepancies, address them immediately so that patients don't have to wait long for a resolution.

3. Offer multiple payment options, such as online bill pays, check or credit card payments, or even installment plans if necessary. This will make it easier for patients to pay their bills without having to go through extra hassle or inconvenience.

4. Stay on top of outstanding balances and follow up with patients who owe money. Don't let unpaid bills go too long without being addressed - this can lead to bad debt and other financial problems down the road.

5. Educate your staff about effective collection techniques so that they can be more proactive in getting paid by patients.

6. Finally, remember that good customer service is key when it comes to collections - always be polite, professional, and helpful whenever you reach out to delinquent account holders.

## CHAPTER TWELVE Avoid these Common Billing and Coding Mistakes

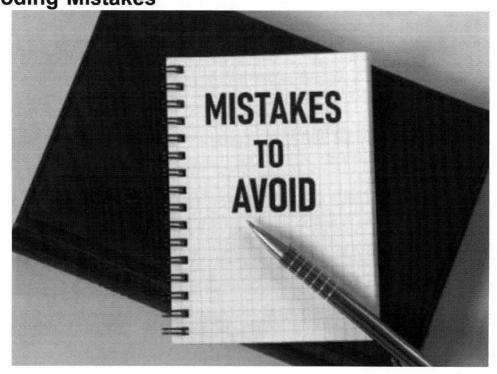

It's a fact that medical billing is no simple job, one reason why the Bureau of Labor Statistics estimates the annual income for a medical billing specialist to be around $56,100. In reality, medical billing is a lot more challenging than just collecting payments from insurance companies. Medical billing specialists must also keep their medical billing department afloat, be ready to handle any unexpected crisis, and be able to code, bill, and manage all medical treatments and services received by their patient base.

However, if you're not prepared with the proper know-how, then you might be making some of these common mistakes that can be very costly for your medical billing company and can even result in a lawsuit. If this is the case, don't get frustrated or start panicking, a medical billing company with experience in coding and billing is your best friend in this situation. Read on to find out some of the common mistakes that can be made when you're billing medical practice.

**Mistake #1:** Not Sending Your Bills to Patients Promptly

Medical billing is one of the most important parts of medical practice, not only for payment but also for the patients and providers to communicate properly. Many medical billing services companies claim that they will send bills immediately to your patients. However, in many cases, this is simply not true. Sometimes, a medical practice can take more than a month to send their bill to the patients. This can cause stress for the patient, the practice as well as the medical biller who has to make sure that they are properly billed and paid for all the services and treatments provided to their patient base. You should also be sending bills to patients promptly, within five days. This is not only important to keep your patient base satisfied, but it will also allow the patient to file claims immediately on their insurance company if they had any claims or bill adjustment that needs to be done. If you're not sending bills to patients promptly, then you should take some time to analyze the patient base of your company.

- ✓ Is your patient base scattered all over the country?
- ✓ Are they receiving bills from multiple medical offices?
- ✓ Does the insurance company require proof that the claim has been sent to the patient?

If these are the cases, then you need to consider upgrading your billing platform.

**Mistake #2:** Not Sending Bills That Have An Effective Date

Medical billing can get complicated and confusing for many medical practices when it comes to sending their bills to the patient. Many medical offices and practices include the date of service, date of billing, date of visit, date of the visit that's being billed, or any other relevant date. Your practice should focus on sending their bill on the date that it's being billed. If your practice has patients who were treated in multiple medical offices and then they all come to you, then they will all get bills at the same time. You'll need to combine all the services provided to your patient based on a single date. You should also be making sure that your patients are able to file claims with their insurance company when the bill is being sent. If you're sending bills that have effective dates, then you should have a patient portal where you can have a system that will notify your patient base if there are any problems with their insurance coverage or claims. Many patient portals allow patients to file claims and make changes to their health coverage. In the case that the patient portal is not properly built or does not notify patients about any insurance coverage issues or bill adjustments, then you should consider upgrading to a medical billing platform that is built with the latest coding techniques and features.

**Mistake #3:** Not Sending Bills That Include the Services and Treatments Provided to Your Patient Base

Just because you're sending your bills to your patient base promptly doesn't mean that you can't make any mistakes in your billings. The common mistake that you might make when it comes to billing is that you're not sending your bills with all the services provided to your patient base. If you're not providing all the services for which the patient paid in their billing statement, then you might want to consider sending it again. Your patient might need some extra clarification to understand what exactly they received and paid for. There's nothing wrong with being a perfectionist. It's just better to have a medical billing company that you can rely on to provide a bill that is concise and includes all the services and treatments that you provided to your patient base. If your billing team is finding it difficult to bill your patient base, then consider a full-time medical biller or a billing professional who can analyze your patient base thoroughly to identify potential issues and then adjust the billing process. This can help your billing team to become more efficient, as well as to make sure that they are providing you with a bill that contains all the services and treatments provided to your patient base.

**Mistake #4:** Improperly Filing Claims for Medications and Other Services

Medication claims are one of the most important parts of medical billing. However, many billing professionals are not filing claims properly. In many cases, your patients who are receiving their medication prescription or medical services might ask you to file a claim for them. If the patients are not properly filing their medication claims, then you need to make sure that you're informing them immediately and sending them the claims so they can get reimbursed. If you're not, then you need to consider upgrading your billing software.

A lot of billing services that claim to offer medication claims might not provide their customers with the ability to send claims. You should also make sure that the pharmaceutical claims are in accordance with the requirements of your patients' insurance companies. If you're not sending your patient's medication claims, then you should be sending them to their pharmacy. If your patient asks you to bill their insurance company for the medications that they're receiving, then you need to make sure that you're following the requirements that their insurance provider has. Many medication claims need to be approved and reimbursed by the insurance company, so you should always be sending the medication claims to your pharmacy and asking them to approve them. The pharmacy should be approving these claims within 7 to 10 business days.

**Mistake #5:** Not Using the Best Coding and Billing Software

Many medical offices and practices rely on medical billing software when it comes to coding and billing their patients. If you're not using the best medical billing software in the market, then you're going to end up making mistakes when it comes to coding and billing. The medical billing software should be able to perform both coding and billing, which means that it should be able to bill the patient and code the medication claims properly. The best medical billing software in the market will be able to provide the following services:

✓ **Ease of use** - The software should be easy to navigate, with a simple user interface.

✓ Billing and invoicing - A good medical billing software should allow you to generate bills and invoices for your patients. This will help you get paid quickly and efficiently.

✓ **Tracking payments** - The software should also track payments, so you can keep tabs on how much money you're owed and when payments are due.

✓ **Generating reports** - The software should also generate reports, so you can see how your business is doing financially and identify areas where improvements can be made.

✓ **Patient management** - The software should help manage your patients' information, such as contact details, insurance info, etc.). This will make it easier to keep track of everything related to each patient's care).

If you're not using the best medical billing software in the market, then you might be coding and billing incorrectly. However, there is no reason to get frustrated, as there are many medical billers who are able to provide their customers with the best medical billing services that are on the market. In case you're coding and billing incorrectly, then you should consider upgrading your billing software.

## Top Billing and Coding Tips from the Experts

Whether you are new to the field or are looking to grow as a professional, knowing some expert tips can improve your medical billing or coding career. Read on to learn more! Here are some tips to help you be successful in your role:

**For medical coders**

1) Stay up to date with the latest coding updates. The ICD-10 code set was updated in 2022, so it's important to make sure you are familiar with the latest changes. The American Health Information Management Association (AHIMA) offers online courses and other resources to help you keep up with the latest coding updates.

2) Use reference materials wisely. There are many reference materials available for medical coders, but it's important not to rely on them too heavily. Each diagnosis or procedure has its unique code, so you must understand the documentation provided by healthcare providers in order to accurately assign codes. AHIMA offers an online course called "Medical Coding and Reimbursement Courses," which teaches how to accurately interpret paper records and assign appropriate codes using ICD-10 guidelines.

The National Cancer Institute also offers a free online course called "Introduction To Coding And billing For Cancer Care." which provides an overview of cancer diagnosis and treatment procedures as well as information on how they should be coded using ICD-10 guidelines.

3) Join professional organizations like AHIMA or AAPC. These organizations offer networking opportunities, continuing education courses, certification programs, and more!

**For medical billers**

1. Get certified. The best way to start your career as a medical biller is by getting certified. Certification shows that you have the necessary skills and knowledge to do the job correctly. There are several different certifications available, so choose one that fits your needs and interests.

2. Stay up-to-date with changes in the industry. The medical billing industry is constantly changing, so billers need to stay up-to-date with new regulations and procedures. Subscribe to newsletters, read trade magazines, or attend conferences and webinars in order to stay current on the latest trends in this field.

3. Develop strong computer skills. Medical billing is largely done online these days, so billers need to have strong computer skills. Be familiar with common software programs used in this field such as Microsoft Office Suite and electronic health record (EHR) systems. Additionally, know how to use search engines and other internet resources effectively when researching specific billing issues.

4. Get experience working with insurance companies. Most insurance companies now require electronic submissions of bills, so having experience submitting bills electronically will give you an advantage over other job applicants. You can gain this type of experience by working as a claims processor or accounts receivable representative at a doctor's office or hospital before making the switch to medical billing

5. Become familiar with ICD - 10 codes. One of the most challenging aspects of being a medical biller is accurately decoding services using ICD - 10 codes. This code set has replaced ICD - 9 codes since, so if you want to be successful in this career field, you need to learn these new codes inside out

6. Understand CPT coding. Another critical skill for medical billers is understanding CPT (Current Procedural Terminology) coding. This coder system provides physicians with a standard language for describing the services they provide patients. Billers must understand what each code means in order not only to submit accurate bills but also to receive appropriate payments from insurers.

7. Be prepared for challenges. As mentioned earlier, the medical billing industry is constantly evolving which can lead to unanticipated challenges for those working in this field.

So whether you are just starting on your journey towards becoming a certified medical coder/biller or are already working within this field – these tips from experts should give you some guidance on what it takes to achieve success!

# CONCLUSION

Billing and coding is a process that is used to track, manage, and bill for medical services. It can be a complex process, but it is important to understand what billing and coding entail in order to ensure that you are getting the most out of your healthcare.

The first step in billing and coding is understanding the codes that are used to describe medical procedures. These codes are standardized by the International Classification of Diseases (ICD), which covers all aspects of healthcare from diagnosis to procedure codes. There are thousands of these codes, so billers and coders need to have a comprehensive understanding of them.

Once the appropriate codes have been selected, they must be translated into specific charges for each service provided. This involves calculating how much time was spent on each procedure, as well as any associated supplies or medications used. The charges generated by this process make up the patient's billable visit amount.

It should be noted that not all services provided during a visit will necessarily generate charges - some may be considered covered under insurance plans or other government programs like Medicare or Medicaid.

This means that proper billing and coding require an understanding not only of ICD-10-CM code sets but also of insurance plan benefits structures. Once all these details have been accounted for, it falls on the coder's shoulders then submit claims correctly formatted so they can get paid quickly!

There is no doubt that this billing and coding guidebook can be a valuable resource for healthcare professionals. However, it is important to remember that this guidebook should not be used as the only source of information when billing and coding patients. The guidebook should be used in conjunction with other resources, such as official coding manuals from the American Medical Association (AMA) and other governing bodies.

Finally, always use caution when interpreting information. If there is any doubt about how a particular code should be applied, seek clarification from an expert before submitting claims for payment.

Made in the USA
Monee, IL
11 December 2024

73050664R00061